# Weight Training For Complete Beginners

Emiliano C. López

All rights reserved. Copyright © 2023 Emiliano C. López

# COPYRIGHT © 2023 Emiliano C. López

All rights reserved.

No part of this book must be reproduced, stored in a retrieval system, or shared by any means, electronic, mechanical, photocopying, recording, or otherwise, without written permission from the publisher.

Every precaution has been taken in the preparation of this book; still the publisher and author assume no responsibility for errors or omissions. Nor do they assume any liability for damages resulting from the use of the information contained herein.

**Legal Notice:**

This book is copyright protected and is only meant for your individual use. You are not allowed to amend, distribute, sell, use, quote or paraphrase any of its part without the written consent of the author or publisher.

# Introduction

This book is a comprehensive guide that delves into the scientific principles, techniques, and strategies behind effective weight training. This guide is a valuable resource for individuals seeking to optimize their strength training routines, improve muscle growth, and enhance their overall fitness.

The guide begins by introducing fundamental training principles that lay the foundation for successful weight training. It covers crucial aspects such as exercise selection, progressive overload, training volume, frequency, repetition ranges, and intensity thresholds. These principles are explained in detail, providing readers with a clear understanding of their importance in achieving desired fitness outcomes.

The concept of training to failure is explored, along with insights into how rest intervals play a role in optimizing workout performance and recovery. The guide goes beyond weight training to discuss concurrent training, which involves combining resistance training with other forms of exercise for a holistic fitness approach.

High-intensity interval training (HIIT) is highlighted as a popular method for improving cardiovascular fitness while complementing weight training routines. Proper warm-up techniques are also emphasized to prevent injuries and enhance workout effectiveness.

A significant portion of the guide is dedicated to "The Big Five Lifts," focusing on key compound exercises that target multiple muscle groups. These exercises, including the bench press, shoulder press, pull-ups, deadlifts, and squats, are broken down with detailed instructions, allowing readers to perform them safely and effectively.

The guide delves into various training methods such as the 10 × 3 method, German Volume Training, pyramid training, reverse pyramid training, drop sets, and cluster sets. It also provides an exploration of periodization, an essential concept in training that involves planned variations in intensity, volume, and exercise selection over specific time periods.

Dietary principles are also covered, addressing topics like calories, energy balance, metabolism, protein, carbohydrates, fats, meal frequency, timing, and post-workout nutrition. The guide explores the concept of intermittent fasting and its potential impact on muscle growth.

Supplements play a role in many fitness routines, and the guide provides insights into popular supplements such as creatine monohydrate, whey protein, branched-chain amino acids, glutamine, caffeine, and beta-alanine.

Training templates are provided for individuals at different training levels, including untrained, recreationally trained, and highly trained. These templates offer structured workout plans tailored to specific fitness goals and experiences.

The guide concludes with loading recommendations and notes on the provided training programs, ensuring that readers have a comprehensive understanding of how to effectively implement the techniques and principles discussed throughout the guide.

Overall, this is an invaluable resource for fitness enthusiasts, athletes, and anyone seeking evidence-based insights into weight training techniques, nutrition, supplementation, and program design. With its detailed explanations, practical advice, and scientific foundation, this guide serves as a comprehensive reference for those looking to optimize their weight training journey.

# Contents

1. TRAINING PRINCIPLES ............................................................................................ 1
    1.1 EXERCISE SELECTION ................................................................................ 2
    1.2 PROGRESSIVE OVERLOAD ......................................................................... 3
    1.3 TRAINING VOLUME .................................................................................... 4
    1.4 TRAINING FREQUENCY ............................................................................. 5
    1.5 REPETITION RANGES .................................................................................. 7
    1.6 INTENSITY THRESHOLDS .......................................................................... 9
    1.7 TRAINING TO FAILURE ............................................................................. 10
    1.8 REST INTERVALS ....................................................................................... 12
    1.9 CONCURRENT TRAINING ........................................................................ 14
    1.10 HIGH-INTENSITY INTERVAL TRAINING ............................................. 16
    1.11 WARMING UP ............................................................................................. 18
2. THE BIG FIVE LIFTS ............................................................................................... 19
    2.1 BENCH PRESS .............................................................................................. 20
    2.2 SHOULDER PRESS ...................................................................................... 21
    2.3 PULL-UPS ...................................................................................................... 22
    2.4 DEADLIFTS .................................................................................................. 24
    2.5 SQUATS ......................................................................................................... 25
3. POPULAR TRAINING METHODS ......................................................................... 27
    3.1 THE 10 × 3 METHOD ................................................................................... 28
    3.2 GERMAN VOLUME TRAINING ................................................................ 29
    3.3 PYRAMID TRAINING ................................................................................. 31
    3.4 REVERSE PYRAMID TRAINING .............................................................. 32
    3.5 DROP SETS ................................................................................................... 33

- 3.6 CLUSTER SETS ................................................................ 34
4. PERIODIZATION ................................................................ 36
  - 4.1 PERIODIZATION BASICS ................................................ 37
  - 4.2 PERIODIZATION THEORY ............................................... 39
  - 4.3 TRAINING CYCLES ........................................................ 41
  - 4.4 TAPER STRATEGIES ...................................................... 42
  - 4.5 LINEAR PERIODIZATION ................................................. 44
  - 4.6 REVERSE-LINEAR PERIODIZATION .................................. 46
  - 4.7 NON-LINEAR PERIODIZATION ......................................... 47
  - 4.8 DAILY UNDULATING PERIODIZATION ............................... 48
  - 4.9 BLOCK PERIODIZATION ................................................. 49
  - 4.10 THE CONJUGATE SYSTEM ............................................ 50
  - 4.11 AUTOREGULATION ..................................................... 51
  - 4.12 WHICH PERIODIZATION MODEL IS BEST? ...................... 54
5. DIET PRINCIPLES ............................................................. 56
  - 5.1 CALORIES .................................................................... 57
  - 5.2 ENERGY BALANCE ....................................................... 58
  - 5.3 METABOLISM ............................................................... 59
  - 5.4 CALCULATING YOUR CALORIE REQUIREMENTS ............... 61
  - 5.5 PROTEIN ..................................................................... 64
  - 5.6 CARBOHYDRATES ........................................................ 65
  - 5.7 FATS ........................................................................... 67
  - 5.8 MEAL FREQUENCY ...................................................... 68
  - 5.9 MEAL TIMING ............................................................... 70
  - 5.10 POST-WORKOUT NUTRITION ........................................ 72
  - 5.11 HYDRATION ............................................................... 74
6. INTERMITTENT FASTING .................................................. 75

- 6.1 OVERVIEW OF INTERMITTENT FASTING ............................................. 76
- 6.2 INTERMITTENT FASTING AND MUSCLEGROWTH ........................... 77
- 7. SUPPLEMENTS ................................................................................................ 79
  - 7.1 CREATINE MONOHYDRATE ................................................................. 80
  - 7.2 WHEY PROTEIN ........................................................................................ 82
  - 7.3 BRANCHED-CHAIN AMINO ACIDS .................................................... 83
  - 7.4 GLUTAMINE .............................................................................................. 84
  - 7.5 CAFFEINE ................................................................................................... 85
  - 7.6 BETA-ALANINE ........................................................................................ 86
- 8. TRAINING TEMPLATES .............................................................................. 87
  - 8.1 UNTRAINED .............................................................................................. 88
  - 8.2 RECREATIONALLY TRAINED .............................................................. 91
  - 8.3 HIGHLY TRAINED ................................................................................... 96
  - 8.4 LOADING RECOMMENDATIONS ..................................................... 101
  - 8.6 NOTES ON THE PROGRAMS .............................................................. 103
- CLOSING STATEMENTS ................................................................................... 104
- GLOSSARY ............................................................................................................ 105

# 1. TRAINING PRINCIPLES

# 1.1 EXERCISE SELECTION

Most weight-training exercises can be divided into two categories: "compound" exercises and "isolation" exercises. Compound exercises (or multi-joint exercises) refer to exercises that stress multiple joints or major muscle groups, whereas isolation exercises stress one joint or major muscle group (1). For instance, a biceps curl only requires your elbow joint to move, whereas a bench press requires both your shoulder joints and your elbow joints to move. In regard to maximizing muscle and strength development, an emphasis should be placed on compound exercises (2, 3) with isolation exercises kept secondary. There are a few reasons for this.

First, performing movements that require the use of multiple joints will work more muscle groups than isolation movements. If we go back to our previous example, we see that the biceps curl primarily works the biceps (one muscle group), whereas the bench press works the chest, shoulders, and triceps. Then if we look at a compound movement like the squat, the difference is even more glaring, considering squats are said to activate over 200 muscles (4). In this regard, compound exercises provide a more efficient way to train the body when compared to isolation movements (5).

Second, compound exercises generally allow you to move more weight than isolation exercises (6). Squats are a great example of this, as they allow you to move far more weight than, say, a leg extension would. Considering this point, many experts suggest that compound exercises may be more suitable for strength development than isolation exercises (2).

## 1.2 PROGRESSIVE OVERLOAD

Progressive overload is the number-one determinant of gaining size and strength. This principle entails progressively overloading the body with stress that it is not accustomed to dealing with (7). In our case, this can mean making the body lift an amount of weight that it is not used to. By doing so, the body will realize that it might have to lift the same amount of weight another time, so it prepares itself by improving neural adaptations needed for force production (8) as well as increasing muscle size (9).

Importantly, adhering to this principle does not mean you must lift heavier weights every week or every training session to overload the body. Another way to accomplish overload is to progressively increase the volume of your training (via more sets or repetitions per set) within reasonable limits (1).

# 1.3 TRAINING VOLUME

Training volume can be defined in two ways. First, volume can refer to the amount of sets × the amount of repetitions performed (1). The other way to define volume is "volume load," which is calculated as the number of sets × the number of repetitions × the load lifted (10). Many researchers prefer to use volume load when discussing training volume since it is generally the best indicator of work done in a training session (3).

While some research suggests otherwise (11–16), the majority of studies show higher training volumes (via more sets) to be more effective for strength gains than lower volumes (17–29). In fact, a meta-analysis by Krieger (30) demonstrated that multiple-set training resulted in 48% greater strength gains than single-set training.

In regard to muscle growth, research has demonstrated a dose-response relationship between the number of sets performed and the magnitude of muscle growth (31–33). These findings are supported by evidence that shows that higher training volumes produce greater elevations in muscle protein synthesis (34–36).

In this training program, the volume will be predicated on what phase of training you are in. For example, the volume in the "Untrained" phase is far less than the volume in the "Highly Trained" phase. This is important because to continually progress over the long term, you must gradually increase your training volume (37).

Furthermore, it is important to note that volume can be looked at in a few different ways. Specifically, there is the training volume of an individual training session, and the amount of volume performed throughout the week. Some strength and conditioning experts prefer to look at training volume as a weekly variable rather than the result of a single training session (32).

# 1.4 TRAINING FREQUENCY

A popular notion within the fitness community is that it is best to "smash" each muscle group in a training session and then allow it a full week to recover before training it again. This notion probably stems from the fact that most bodybuilders train each muscle group once per week (38). Unfortunately, this has led many lifters to believe that if they mimic such a routine, they will achieve maximal results. This may not be the case.

A recent meta-analysis by Schoenfeld and colleagues (39) demonstrated that training each muscle group 2–3 times per week was more effective for muscle growth versus training each muscle group just 1 time per week. This is in line with Schoenfeld's previous study on the topic (40), which demonstrated that training each muscle group 3 times per week produced greater muscle growth versus training each muscle group once per week, even though weekly training volume was equated.

Interestingly, an unpublished study out of Norway (41) demonstrated that training each muscle group 6 times per week produced greater muscular adaptations in elite powerlifters versus training each muscle group 3 times per week (with weekly volume equated between groups). While these findings are certainly intriguing, drawing conclusions off of one unpublished study would be presumptuous.

The benefit behind higher training frequencies might be due to protein synthesis elevations, which have been shown to plateau around 36 hours following training in experienced lifters (42). Therefore, by continually training each muscle group at a high frequency, this will continually "spike" the protein synthesis response, which would theoretically result in more muscle growth (43).

## RECOMMENDATIONS

Given the current evidence, it is recommended that each muscle group be trained a minimum of twice per week to optimize muscle growth (39).

Whether training each muscle group 3 times per week is superior to twice per week requires further investigation (39).

As a side note, it is important to realize that the higher your training frequency during the week, the lower the volume of each training session must be to prevent overtraining. For instance, if you routinely perform 12 sets per muscle group once per week and decide to increase your training frequency to 3 times per week, it would be foolish to perform 12 sets per muscle group 3 times per week (translating to 36 sets per week).

Rather than doing this, divide your weekly number of sets by the amount of training sessions you will be performing throughout the week. In this scenario, the lifter will perform 4 sets each training session, for a total of 12 sets per week. Over time, the lifter can gradually increase the number of sets performed per training session to continue their progression.

# 1.5 REPETITION RANGES

It is commonly recommended to train within a certain repetition range that corresponds with your goal. Specifically, some experts will advise to train in a 1–3 repetition range for power, a 3–8 repetition range for strength, and a 8–15 repetition range for hypertrophy (6). While lower repetitions appear to be necessary for maximizing strength and power, training for hypertrophy may not require a specific repetition range at all.

A study by Schoenfeld et al. (44) compared the effects of a typical powerlifting set–rep scheme (7 sets of 3 reps) to a traditional bodybuilding-style scheme (3 sets of 10 reps). Since the lifters in the powerlifting rep range were able to move more weight (given the lower reps), this resulted in both groups training with an equal amount of volume load. Surprisingly, after 8 weeks of study, both groups achieved an equal amount of muscle growth. These results are in agreement with a study by Klemp et al. (45), which also showed similar muscle growth between a low-repetition group and a high-repetition group when volume load was equated. Therefore, the notion that there is a specific repetition range conducive to hypertrophy appears to be misguided.

Furthermore, while the aforementioned studies equated volume load between groups, a subsequent study by Schoenfeld and colleagues (46)—which did not equate for volume load—produced even more intriguing findings. In this study, the researchers compared the effects of a "high-load" condition (8–12 reps per set) to a "low-load" condition (25–35 reps per set). All of the participants were experienced lifters, therefore negating the possibility of a "novice effect."

After 8 weeks of study, both groups achieved a similar amount of muscle growth. It is important to note, however, that the low-load group trained with a much greater amount of volume than the high-load group, which could explain the results from the training. Regardless, this study further demonstrates that there is no optimal repetition range for hypertrophy, and that training anywhere from 1–35+ repetitions per set can produce significant gains in muscle growth, given an adequate training volume.

As mentioned previously, while specific repetition ranges will not have a big impact on muscle growth (if your total volume is sufficient), they appear to have an impact on strength. While the study by Klemp et al. did not find differences in hypertrophy or strength gains between the high and low-rep groups, the majority of research indicates greater strength gain potential with lower repetitions compared to higher ones (44, 46, 47).

# 1.6 INTENSITY THRESHOLDS

As just discussed, lifters can experience ample muscle growth when training in repetition ranges as high as 35 per set. These findings have lead researchers to wonder what the minimum intensity threshold is for maximizing hypertrophic gains (48). While it is commonly suggested that a minimum intensity threshold of around 70% of your 1 rep max (1RM) is required to maximize muscle growth (49, 50), this notion has been challenged by low-load training studies. Specifically, when comparing the effects of a low-load condition (training with 20–30% of a 1RM) to a high-load condition (75–80% 1RM), numerous studies have demonstrated similar muscle growth between conditions (51–55).

The mechanism behind why equivalent results can occur between such different loading intensities is unclear. It has been suggested that since the low-load groups trained their sets to muscular failure, the onset of fatigue would result in maximal motor unit recruitment (56, 57), thus explaining the similar muscle growth to the high-load conditions. Other researchers speculate that the similar outcomes in hypertrophy are the result of the low-load groups increasing the size of their type I muscle fibers (58). Considering these fiber types are characterized as "fatigue resistant," it is logical to presume that a longer time under tension would result in the maximal stimulation of these fibers (59). Recent evidence out of Russia supports this viewpoint, as studies have demonstrated greater growth of the type I muscle fibers through performing high repetitions with light loads (60, 61). This is in contrast to heavier load training, where it was found that the type II fibers experienced greater growth.

While further research is needed to confirm the exact mechanism at work, it is clear that low-load training can induce profound muscle growth (62). This may serve well for individuals who prefer to train in higher repetition ranges. It should be noted, however, that if maximal muscle growth is the goal, it might be beneficial to train in a spectrum of repetition ranges to maximize the growth of the type I and type II muscle fibers (59).

# 1.7 TRAINING TO FAILURE

As we just saw, training to failure may be necessary for maximal muscle growth when training with very light loads. However, when it comes to training with more conventional loads (over 70% 1RM), training to failure may not be necessary.

Advocates of failure training say that pushing the muscle to exhaustion during a set is necessary to maximize motor unit recruitment (63), which will maximize strength gains (64). Contrasting this viewpoint however, Sundstrup and colleagues (65) demonstrated that training to failure was unnecessary for maximizing motor unit recruitment when using a conventional intensity threshold.

Furthermore, while some researchers advocate training to failure as a means to maximize muscle and strength gains, others state that it may be detrimental. A common criticism of failure training is that it makes it difficult for the lifter to sustain a certain workload over subsequent sets because of the dramatic onset of fatigue during the first set (66). In other words, given that the body is pushed to its limit during the first set, it may not be strong enough to sustain a given intensity within a specific repetition range over the next work sets, thus impairing training volume. Another criticism of failure training is that it may increase the risk of injuries and overtraining (66).

Studies on the topic have been divided. Some have shown an advantage of failure training for strength gains (67), whereas others show no advantage (68). A recent meta-analysis by Davies and colleagues (66) demonstrated that training to failure does not result in favorable strength outcomes compared to non-failure training.

## RECOMMENDATIONS

Given the potential issues with training to failure during conventional loading, it appears to be an unwarranted strategy for maximizing training adaptations. However, for those who wish to use failure training, there are a few ways to incorporate it into your routine while minimizing the drawbacks that it presents.

First, rather than training to failure on every set, it would be more beneficial to reserve training to failure for your final set. This way, you get your training volume in for the session while fully exhausting the muscles during the final set, which will not detract from your total training volume.

Another option is to reserve failure training for certain weeks of training (for instance, 1 or 2 weeks out of each month) to allow variation to be incorporated into your workouts. While these are viable options for including failure training into your routine, lifters should closely monitor the impact that it has on their ability to recover.

# 1.8 REST INTERVALS

A frequently misunderstood aspect of weight training is the optimal rest interval length between sets to maximize adaptations from training. It is generally believed that if hypertrophy is the goal, then short rest intervals (1 minute) are best, because this maximizes growth hormone secretion (69). While this is indeed true (70–73), research has suggested that growth hormone has no effect on muscle anabolism in healthy individuals (74–84). Furthermore, when you analyze the studies that compare rest interval durations between sets, it becomes apparent that shorter rests may not be optimal for muscle and strength gains.

In a review of the literature, Henselmans and Schoenfeld (85) did not find one study that showed an advantage of short rest intervals over long rest intervals for promoting muscle growth. Following this review however, a study by Villanueva and colleagues (86) showed that 1 minute rest intervals were superior for muscle and strength gains in elderly men compared to 4 minute rest intervals.

Contrasting these findings, Schoenfeld and colleagues (87) compared the effects of 1 minute rest intervals to 3 minute rest intervals on muscle size and strength over an 8 week training period. At the end of the study, the long rest interval group achieved greater muscle and strength gains than the short rest group. These findings have been supported by research showing that shorter rest intervals impair protein synthesis elevations following strength training (88).

Now, while a limited amount of research has shown an advantage of shorter rest intervals compared to longer ones, the majority of evidence indicates that longer rest intervals are superior for muscle and strength gains. The reasoning behind this may be due to training volume. Common sense tells us that the shorter you rest between sets, the more fatigued you will be going into the next set. This will inevitably result in fewer repetitions performed per set, which will decrease training volume (89–94). Given the importance of training volume for muscle growth, hindering it by using short rest intervals may be detrimental to long-term muscle gains.

## RECOMMENDATIONS

Given the totality of evidence, using short rest intervals between sets appears to be unnecessary, and may in fact be detrimental to muscle and strength gains. Therefore, it is recommended that rest interval durations last at least 3 minutes to allow for an optimal sustainability of training volume (94).

# 1.9 CONCURRENT TRAINING

In addition to its benefits on cardiovascular health (95), endurance training has been shown to enhance cognition (96–103), improve brain health (104, 105), and reduce depression (106–118). Furthermore, endurance training is necessary for athletes who require both aerobic fitness in addition to strength and power. Therefore, many athletes will integrate endurance training into their lifting regimen, a practice known as "concurrent training." While endurance training can provide numerous health benefits as mentioned above, whether it is beneficial for someone looking to maximize muscle and strength gains remains controversial.

## THE INTERFERENCE EFFECT

While some research has demonstrated no negative effects of endurance training on muscle and strength gains (119–131), other research has shown endurance training to be detrimental to at least one of these goals (132–141). This is thought to be due to an "interference effect" (142, 143) whereby muscle and strength adaptations cannot be maximized because of the divergent nature of endurance and strength training (144).

## MODALITY OF ENDURANCE TRAINING

It should be noted that in the majority of studies comparing strength training to concurrent training, the usual methods of endurance exercise are either in the form of running or cycling. Researchers have speculated whether the type of endurance exercise performed can impact the interference effect on muscle and strength gains (145). Fortunately, a meta-analysis by Wilson and colleagues (146) revealed that while running caused significant decrements in muscle and strength gains when performed concurrently with strength training, cycling did not. The researchers speculate that this may be because cycling is less damaging to the leg muscles than running, given that cycling is primarily a concentric movement compared to running, which has a high eccentric component.

Furthermore, the researchers suggest that endurance training of shorter durations and higher intensities may produce less of an interference effect with strength training compared to longer duration endurance training.

## RECOMMENDATIONS

Given these findings, it is recommended that if muscle and strength gains are the primary goal, endurance training should be kept to a minimum to avoid any possible interference in maximizing these attributes. Athletes who require both strength as well as endurance are advised to emphasize cycling over running, as well as high-intensity interval training (HIIT) over steady-state cardio (146). In addition to HIIT possibly mitigating the interference effect to strength training, research has shown it to be a highly efficient strategy for fat loss and aerobic fitness (147). We discuss this next.

# 1.10 HIGH-INTENSITY INTERVAL TRAINING

## HOW IT WORKS

High-intensity interval training (HIIT) consists of short bursts of high-intensity output (such as "all out" sprints) followed by a rest between sets (148). An example of this would be sprinting as hard as possible for 30 seconds followed by 1 minute of jogging or walking. This process is then repeated several times for a given number of sets. It is important to note that HIIT can be incorporated into many aerobic activities, including cycling, swimming, and cross-country skiing. Its mainstream emergence as an effective alternative for aerobic training is the result of numerous studies demonstrating its potency for promoting fat loss and aerobic fitness with very short workouts.

## THE EFFICIENCY OF HIIT

To illustrate this point, Gibala and colleagues (149) compared the effects of six HIIT sessions to steady-state cardio over a 2 week period. The HIIT group gradually increased their workload to 6 sets of 30 second "all out" sprints on an exercise bicycle, followed by 4 minutes of rest between sets. The steady-state cardio group performed 90–120 minutes of continuous cycling. At the end of the study, both groups saw similar improvements in their time trial performance. What was astonishing, however, was that the HIIT group performed significantly less total work than the steady-state group during the experimental period. As the authors note, the HIIT group trained for a total of 2.5 hours during the 2 week training period, compared to the 10.5 hours of training time for the steady-state group.

In regard to fat loss, a recent meta-analysis (150) found that HIIT was as effective as steady-state cardio for improving body composition, however, HIIT required 40% less training time than steady-state cardio.

## THE EFFECTIVENESS OF HIIT

In addition to being extremely time efficient, a meta-analysis by Milanović and colleagues (151) revealed HIIT to be superior for increasing aerobic capacity (VO2 max) versus steady-state cardio. These findings suggest that even though HIIT is more time efficient than steady-state cardio, it may even produce greater improvements in aerobic fitness.

## SETTING UP A HIIT PROGRAM

When setting up an appropriate training structure with HIIT, a 1:1 work-to-rest ratio is recommended for athletes, whereas the general population may be better off with a 1:2 work-to-rest ratio (152). For those who are less fit, a 1:4 work to rest ratio may be employed until greater fitness levels are achieved (152).

**EXAMPLES:**

### 1:4 Work-to-Rest Ratio (Beginner)

10 second sprint (90–100% max effort) followed by a 40 second jog.

Repeat 5 times.

### 1:2 Work-to-Rest Ratio (Intermediate)

20 second sprint (90–100% max effort) followed by a 40 second jog.

Repeat 5–8 times.

### 1:1 Work-to-Rest Ratio (Advanced)

30 second sprint (90–100% max effort) followed by a 30 second jog.

Repeat 8–10 times.

# 1.11 WARMING UP

Contrary to popular belief, it may not be wise to perform lengthy stretching sessions before a strength workout. This was demonstrated in a review by Behm and colleagues (153), which showed that static stretching prior to training resulted in impaired strength performance. Furthermore, studies have shown significant reductions in training volume when stretching was performed prior to training (154, 155).

## RECOMMENDATIONS

Given these findings, it appears that stretching before a strength-training bout may be unwise. Rather than doing this, it would be better to increase blood flow into the muscles, as this will "prime" them for handling heavy weights. A good option is to perform 5–10 minutes of cycling followed by a few warm-up sets for the given body part you are training. This can include lifting the bar for a high number of repetitions or performing a few sets of bodyweight exercises prior to your heavy work sets. This type of warm-up will be more beneficial to your training given that it will increase body temperature, which has been shown to positively affect power output (156).

# 2. THE BIG FIVE LIFTS

## 2.1 BENCH PRESS

Undoubtedly a very popular exercise for recreational lifters, the bench press is a great movement for the chest, triceps, and shoulders. An important note to remember is that for chest days, the term "bench press" can mean either bench pressing with a barbell or with dumbbells. Interestingly, pressing with dumbbells has taken over as the popular option to train the chest because of the slightly greater range of motion that it allows. Furthermore, pressing with dumbbells allows your wrists to maintain a more natural position than pressing with a barbell does.

On the other hand, using a barbell enables you to use more weight than dumbbells do (157). As we discussed earlier, using more weight in any exercise can be advantageous for gaining size and strength, but the same could be said for range of motion.

In terms of muscle activation, a study out of Norway (157) revealed that both barbells and dumbbells activated the chest and shoulders to a similar extent. Interestingly, the triceps were activated more with the barbell bench press whereas the biceps were activated more with the dumbbell bench press.

## 2.2 SHOULDER PRESS

Being a compound movement that allows you to use a lot of weight, the shoulder press is a great choice for adding size to your shoulders. There are several options when performing this exercise. Some lifters elect to do them standing, while others are more comfortable doing them seated. Furthermore, the shoulder press can be performed with either barbells or dumbbells. Interestingly, another Norwegian study (158) demonstrated that standing shoulder presses activated the shoulders to a greater extent than seated presses. In addition, dumbbells appeared to be more effective than barbells for shoulder activation.

## 2.3 PULL-UPS

One of the most effective upper body exercises you can do, pull-ups allow you to move a lot of weight (159) and work a lot of muscles. Furthermore, pull-ups are categorized as a "closed-chain movement," meaning that the hands are fixed in place while the body moves through space. This is in contrast to open-chain exercises, whereby the body remains stationary and the hands or feet move in space. Interestingly, a study by Prokopy and colleagues (160) showed closed-chain exercises to be more effective for power improvements than open-chain exercises.

### PULL-UPS VERSUS CHIN-UPS

While these terms are sometimes used interchangeably, most fitness practitioners distinguish the term "pull-up" from "chin-up" by the palm grip. Specifically, if your palms are facing out and away from you when gripping the bar, this is referred to as a pull-up. When your palms are facing toward you while gripping the bar, this is a chin-up. While neither movement presents a significant advantage over the other for activating the lats (the large muscles along the sides of your back), the chin-up has been shown to activate the biceps to a greater extent than the pull-up (161).

### HAND PLACEMENT

Certainly one of the major misconceptions in strength-training circles relates to the optimal grip width for performing pull-ups. Many people believe that using a very wide grip placement on the bar will allow you to more effectively activate the lat muscles. While this has been shown to be true for lat pull-downs (162), what is not accounted for is the range of motion. Specifically, research has shown that range of motion has a significant impact on enhancing muscle growth (163, 164). Since a wide hand placement will cause your range of motion to suffer, this may hinder your ability to maximize muscle gains. Given this, it is recommended to use a moderate grip placement that allows for a full range of motion throughout the movement.

## 2.4 DEADLIFTS

Deadlifts are one of the best exercises you can perform for increasing muscle size and strength. They are a very simple exercise because you are essentially just bending down and lifting a bar off the ground. While it may not look as flashy as other movements, this does not take away from its effectiveness. The reasons for this include the vast amount of weight that deadlifts allow you to use, as well as the amount of muscles worked. These include your traps, lower back, abs, obliques, glutes, quads, hamstrings, and forearms.

### PROPER FORM

- For deadlifts, it is best to assume an over-under grip (meaning one hand will grip the bar underhand, while the other grips it overhand). Doing this will ensure that the bar doesn't roll out of your hands during the lift.
- Never bend over and lift the weight with a rounded lower back. A good way to ensure proper back alignment is to keep your chest up and your hips kicked back.
- Stand with the bar as close to your shins as possible before the lift. This will help you in getting the weight up.
- Keep your arms completely straight throughout the movement. Never bend them toward you as if you were trying to curl the weight. Doing this can result in a biceps tear.

# 2.5 SQUATS

Along with deadlifts, squats are largely considered to be a king of muscle builders. This is for good reason, since they are among the best exercises you can do to build your legs and glutes, in addition to increasing overall athleticism.

## PROPER FORM

- The first thing you want to do is ensure that your stance is roughly shoulder-width apart with your toes facing forward or slightly outward (165).
- As with deadlifts, it is important to keep your trunk as rigid as possible throughout the exercise.
- Keep your chest up and your shoulder blades retracted throughout the movement (166).
- Before the descent phase, inhale with about 80% of maximal inhalation and then hold your breath to increase intra-abdominal pressure (165).
- For head alignment, do not look down or up when squatting. Simply keep your head in a neutral position (aligned with the spine) throughout the movement (165).
- The descent phase is initiated by sitting the hips back while maintaining a rigid upper body posture with your chest sticking outward (165).

## BAR PLACEMENT

For bar placement, you have two choices. The first is called a "high bar" squat. This is a squat where the bar rests atop your trapezius muscles, which is the most common form of bar placement.

On the other hand, some people elect to rest the bar farther down their back. This is called a "low bar" squat. This is where the bar is essentially touching the back of the shoulders.

While neither choice is drastically superior to the other, most powerlifters elect to use a low bar placement because it puts the body in a more mechanically efficient position to get the weight up. This will allow you to lift slightly more weight (167).

# 3. POPULAR TRAINING METHODS

## 3.1 THE 10 × 3 METHOD

The 10 × 3 method entails picking a compound exercise and performing 10 sets of 3 repetitions at 80–85% of your 1 rep max. As you can probably tell, this scheme is basically the reverse of a typical 3 × 10 routine that many lifters employ. However, not only does 10 × 3 allow for a greater volume load to be used compared to 3 × 10, the other benefit of this method is the intensity it permits. By training at 80–85% of your 1RM, you are essentially in the "sweet spot" for maximizing strength gains, provided that you have training experience (37). While lower training intensities can promote substantial muscle growth, they are likely not as effective as higher intensities for increasing maximal strength (62).

The final benefit of 10 × 3 is its effect on technique work. Rather than performing 3 or even 5 sets per exercise, 10 × 3 demands that you perform 10 sets. If we take an exercise like the barbell squat, which demands a high level of technique to be proficient at, we see that performing more sets gives you more opportunity to practice technique.

## 3.2 GERMAN VOLUME TRAINING

German Volume Training (GVT, or the 10 set method) was purportedly developed by an Olympic weightlifting coach to increase muscle mass in lifters during the off season (168). The purpose of this training scheme is to manipulate the variables of training volume and metabolic stress to promote muscle growth.

Essentially, GVT entails picking a compound exercise and performing 10 sets of 10 repetitions of that exercise. At about 60–65% of your 1 rep max, the weight used will feel rather light. Increases in weight are only permitted once the lifter can perform all 10 repetitions of each set. To maximize metabolic stress, rest intervals are typically kept short during the workout, at about 60–90 seconds between sets. While the rationale behind this is sound, I personally do not recommend keeping the rest intervals this short since the majority of research demonstrates superior muscle growth with longer rest intervals. If you elect to rest longer between sets, then the weight used may be increased to 65–70% of your 1 rep max.

Given the high amount of volume that this training scheme provides, it is advised that it only be used once you have reached a high level of training status. A recent study (169) demonstrated that a modified GVT protocol was inferior to a 5 × 10 protocol for inducing muscle and strength gains; however, the subjects in the GVT protocol only had an average of 3.5 years of training experience. Given that training volume must progressively increase in conjunction with training status (37), performing higher volume protocols such as GVT may only be beneficial to lifters with very high experience levels.

This notion is supported by a meta-analysis by Peterson and colleagues (170), which demonstrated that athletes require twice the amount of training volume to maximize strength gains compared to non-athletes. According to the effect size data, athletes experience the greatest strength increases when performing 8 sets per muscle group. This is in contrast to non-athletes, who only need 4 sets to achieve maximal strength gains (171). While these findings relate solely to strength and not hypertrophy, it is plausible that highly advanced lifters would benefit more from a GVT protocol (for both hypertrophy and strength) than less experienced lifters.

Importantly, temporary cycles of very high training volumes (i.e., overreaching phases) within a periodized training plan may be beneficial to maximize muscle adaptations. It is crucial, however, that an unloading cycle follows each overreaching phase to offset the possibility of overtraining. We discuss unloading cycles in section 4.3.

## 3.3 PYRAMID TRAINING

A popular training method, pyramid training consists of opening your workout with a moderate weight for a high number of repetitions, then progressively increasing the weight while decreasing the repetitions each set. In other words, you are "pyramiding" up in weight throughout the workout.

One of the benefits of this training method is the safety aspect. By beginning your work sets with a moderate weight for a high number of repetitions, you are allowing your body to essentially "warm-up" within the workout. This will aid your ability to tolerate heavier weights with each subsequent set. An example of a typical pyramid scheme is as follows:

**SET 1:** 15 reps @ 65% 1RM

**SET 2:** 10 reps @ 70% 1RM

**SET 3:** 8 reps @ 75% 1RM

**SET 4:** 5 reps @ 80% 1RM

**SET 5:** 3 reps @ 90% 1RM

## 3.4 REVERSE PYRAMID TRAINING

Reverse pyramid training is simply pyramid training run backward. Rather than beginning the workout with a moderate weight for a high number of repetitions, you begin the workout with the heaviest weight you can handle for a low number of repetitions (after a few warm-up sets). You then continue to pyramid down in weight while increasing the repetitions for each set. An example is shown below:

**SET 1:** 3 reps @ 90% 1RM

**SET 2:** 5 reps @ 80% 1RM

**SET 3:** 8 reps @ 75% 1RM

**SET 4:** 10 reps @ 70% 1RM

**SET 5:** 15 reps @ 65% 1RM

Advocates of this training method state that since the body is the most fresh at the beginning of a workout, it only makes sense to use the heaviest amount of weight at that point. This way, intensity is maximized while each subsequent set is used as a means to "get your volume in" for the training session.

It should go without saying that this training method should never be performed without an adequate warm-up, since beginning your workout with the heaviest weight possible can pose an increased risk of injury.

## 3.5 DROP SETS

A popular training method among bodybuilders, drop sets involve performing a regular work set to muscular failure, and then immediately reducing the weight to allow for more repetitions to be completed until subsequent failure (172). This can be accomplished by having a training partner quickly take a few plates off the barbell once failure has been reached. When training with dumbbells, the lifter can immediately switch to a lighter pair once he or she has reached failure with the initial pair of dumbbells.

It has been suggested that drop sets may induce greater training adaptations through motor unit fatigue (172). Interestingly, a recent study (173) showed that drop set training produced larger effect sizes for muscle growth compared to traditional "straight set" training.

These findings run contrary to a separate study (174), which showed drop set training to be no more effective than traditional training for muscle growth. As the researchers note, however, the choice of measurement used to detect muscle changes was not optimal.

Despite these conflicting findings, drop sets can be an effective strategy for those looking to increase training volume and time under tension during their workouts.

## 3.6 CLUSTER SETS

A recent and intriguing strategy for strength training is the use of cluster sets. A cluster set is essentially a training set with brief rest intervals interspersed within the set. To use a set of 12 repetitions as an example, a traditional set would entail performing the 12 repetitions non-stop followed by a rest interval of a few minutes before going into the next set. With cluster set training, rather than doing 12 repetitions consecutively, these repetitions are broken up with very short rest intervals (10–30 seconds) within the set.

An example would be performing 4 repetitions followed by a short rest 3 times. Another possibility is to divide the set in half by performing 6 repetitions followed by a short rest interval, and then completing the next 6 repetitions. Once the set of 12 is complete, a regular rest interval of a few minutes will commence until the next cluster set.

The following is an example of a basic cluster set workout. It should be noted that cluster sets may be designed in any fashion the lifter deems fit. This may include placing the intra-set rest interval after each repetition, following each 3 repetitions, after each 10 repetitions, and so on.

**CLUSTER SET 1:** $3 \times 5$ (15 second rests within the set)

Rest 3 minutes

**CLUSTER SET 2:** $3 \times 5$ (15 second rests within the set)

Rest 3 minutes

**CLUSTER SET 3:** $3 \times 5$ (15 second rests within the set)

## PURPORTED BENEFITS OF CLUSTER SETS

The rationale behind this training strategy is that the intra-set rest intervals will allow for a greater quality of repetitions to be performed throughout the set (175). This is opposed to traditional sets where no rest is taken in between repetitions, which inevitably leads to muscular fatigue, thus decreasing the quality of lifting at the latter end of the set.

Specifically, proponents of cluster set training suggest that the rest afforded within each set will allow the athlete to lift the weight at maximum velocity, thus increasing power output (175). It has also been suggested that this training style may not be ideal for developing strength and hypertrophy given that muscular fatigue is avoided with cluster set training (175).

Conversely, however, the additional rests within sets allows the lifter to use heavier loads and perform more total repetitions per workout (176). While this would conceivably result in greater muscle and strength gains, more research is needed to determine if this is the case.

When making use of cluster set training, it has been suggested that this method is best reserved for experienced lifters using explosive exercises. For instance, cluster set training may be beneficial for exercises such as power cleans and snatches, which require a great level of technical proficiency (175).

As an important side note, it is recommended that the lifter unload the weight (e.g., by racking the bar) during each intra-set rest interval as opposed to continually bearing the weight throughout the set (176). This will allow for a complete alleviation of tension on the muscles, thus allowing for a higher-quality rest period.

# 4. PERIODIZATION

# 4.1 PERIODIZATION BASICS

### WHAT IS PERIODIZATION?

Periodization can be defined as a cyclic structure of training designed to maximize performance, manage fatigue, and minimize plateaus (177). It works by manipulating training variables such as volume, intensity, frequency, and exercise selection to attain the benefits of each variable at the most opportune time (178).

### THE PURPOSE OF PERIODIZATION

Generally speaking, periodized training programs are designed to best prepare an athlete for an upcoming competition. For instance, they are commonly used by powerlifters to peak in strength for an upcoming meet. Since continuous use of the same loading zone may result in stagnation, periodization allows for structured variation to be incorporated into training, thus resulting in greater adaptations (179–182). This concept has been validated in research, as periodized training has been shown to be more effective for strength gains than non-periodized training (183, 184).

### SHOULD EVERYONE PERIODIZE?

There is prevailing controversy on whether periodization is necessary for novice lifters (185). This is primarily because of a beginner's ability to make rapid strength gains in a linear fashion. Specifically, since most beginners are easily able to progress in size and strength from the novel stimulus of weight training, there would be no need for periodization, as it would only complicate matters. This is why it is advocated that periodization should be reserved for more experienced lifters, since they have greater difficulty achieving muscle and strength gains compared to novice lifters (186).

While the logic behind this thinking is sound, multiple meta-analyses (183, 184) have demonstrated that untrained individuals experience significantly greater strength gains with periodized training compared to non-periodized training. Given this evidence, it appears that lifters of all experience levels can benefit from periodized training plans.

# 4.2 PERIODIZATION THEORY

## GENERAL ADAPTATION SYNDROME

The basis behind periodization originated from Hans Selye's general adaptation syndrome (187–189). This concept states that when an organism is faced with an external stressor, it will experience three stages of reactions:

1. **Alarm reaction:** In this stage, the organism is faced with an external stressor that it is ill equipped to deal with. In regard to weight training, this stage would equate to an amount of training load that the athlete is not used to.
2. **Resistance:** Following the alarm reaction is the stage of resistance. It is during this stage that the organism develops adaptations to handle the stressor. This coincides with an athlete adapting to weight training by increasing his or her muscle size and strength.
3. **Exhaustion:** The final stage of the general adaptation syndrome is the exhaustion stage. According to Selye, an organism cannot continue to tolerate the same stressor forever, which will inevitably result in a deteriorating effect. With weight training, this can result in stagnation or even overtraining. This is why it is recommended to incorporate variation into the training plan to ensure optimal progression.

## FITNESS-FATIGUE MODEL

While periodization's popularity originated through its association with the general adaptation syndrome (190), another model has been proposed to better explain the basis of periodization. The fitness-fatigue model states that when an individual undergoes physical training, both fitness and fatigue aftereffects will accumulate (191).

The model also states that it is the difference between fitness and fatigue that will determine the athlete's readiness to perform. Specifically, if fitness aftereffects greatly outweigh fatigue aftereffects, then the athlete will be in "peak form." On the other hand, if fatigue greatly exceeds fitness, then overtraining may occur (191).

Therefore, the goal of periodization is to maximize fitness aftereffects while minimizing fatigue aftereffects at the most opportune time.

## 4.3 TRAINING CYCLES

When discussing periodization, it is important to understand the terminology used for periodized programs. These terms refer to specific training cycles within the periodized training plan. They include the microcycle, mesocycle, and macrocycle (192).

- **Microcycle**: Generally represents 1 week of training (193). These can be manipulated to incorporate different loading strategies, as seen in daily undulating periodization. Exercise selection can also vary throughout each microcycle if desired.

- **Mesocycle**: Generally represents 1 month of training (193). In linear and reverse-linear periodization models, these training phases are usually characterized by training in a specific loading zone.

- **Macrocycle**: Generally represents 1 year of training (193). Competitions where peak performance must be attained are planned throughout the macrocycle.

- **Taper period:** A taper consists of systematic reductions in training volume for a 1–4 week period to promote peak levels of physical preparedness. These periods are generally implemented before important competitions (194).

- **Unloading cycle:** Similar to taper periods, unloading cycles consist of reduced training loads (either volume, intensity, or both) to promote recovery and adaptation from training. These training cycles generally last 1 week in duration and are implemented at the end of a mesocycle to promote fitness adaptations for the following mesocycle.

It should be noted that substantial variability exists between the lengths of each training cycle (193). Depending on the goals of the athlete, the training cycles may last longer than depicted above, and some may last shorter.

41

## 4.4 TAPER STRATEGIES

Generally speaking, there are three types of taper strategies that can be implemented into a training plan (193, 194):

- **The step taper:** This strategy consists of an abrupt and dramatic reduction in training volume that is kept constant throughout the duration of the taper period. For instance, dropping training volume by 50% and maintaining this volume throughout the taper period (193).

- **The linear taper:** This strategy entails constant decreases in training volume from workout to workout in a linear fashion. For instance, dropping training volume by 5% of the initial value each workout (193).

- **The exponential taper:** This strategy entails decreasing training volume at a rate proportional to its current value (194). For instance, the lifter may decrease his or her volume by 5% of the previous value of the prior training session (193).

### THE MOST EFFECTIVE TAPER STRATEGY

While research has shown the exponential taper to produce optimal results for endurance athletes (195), recommendations specific to strength athletes are lacking. For the purpose of simplicity, it may be beneficial to use a step taper to easily monitor volume reductions. It is recommended that a 30–70% reduction in training volume be implemented during the taper period, with intensity maintained or slightly increased (196).

### TRAINING CESSATION

Another option for lifters who are nearing the end of a training cycle is the use of complete training cessation as opposed to a structured taper. In other words, rather than continuing to train with a reduced training volume, a lifter may completely stop training for a short time period if he or she is feeling particularly worn down. While this represents an alternative strategy to promote recovery and adaptation, it is stressed that training cessation should last no longer than 1 week, as periods longer than this may result in strength decrements (196).

## 4.5 LINEAR PERIODIZATION

Linear periodization is the most basic and traditional form of periodized training. It typically involves progressing from high-volume, low-intensity workouts to lower-volume, higher-intensity workouts (197). The purpose of this periodization model is to gain muscle mass during the high-volume phase, which will best prepare the athlete for increasing strength and power during the following phases (198). Furthermore, lifting technique is increasingly emphasized the closer the athlete gets to a competition.

A basic example of a linear periodization model is shown below. Note the progressive reduction in volume from mesocycle to mesocycle, while training intensity is increased.

| DURATION | SET–REP SCHEME | INTENSITY |
|---|---|---|
| WEEKS: 1–4 | 5 × 12 | 70% |
| WEEKS: 5–8 | 5 × 6 | 80% |
| WEEKS: 9–12 | 5 × 3 | 90% |

It should also be remembered that a high degree of variability exists regarding the durations of each phase as well as the set–rep scheme employed. Furthermore, some strength and conditioning coaches will implement an unloading cycle near the end of each mesocycle to transition the athlete into the next mesocycle (193).

As a side note, while this periodization model is simplest to understand through the term "linear" periodization (given its linear progression from lower to higher intensities), this is a misnomer given that training phases are incorporated in a wave-like (non-linear) manner throughout the macrocycle (177). This is why some experts refer to this model as "traditional" or "classic" periodization, which does allow for some variation to take place even within the microcycle. For the purpose of simplicity, we will use the term linear periodization to describe this model.

## 4.6 REVERSE-LINEAR PERIODIZATION

Reverse-linear periodization is virtually identical to linear periodization, with the sole difference being that the scheme is run backward. Rather than progressively reducing training volume while increasing intensity, this model reduces intensity while increasing volume (199). Below is a basic example of how one might set up a reverse-linear periodization protocol. Remember that a high degree of variability can exist between duration lengths and repetition schemes depending on the lifter's goals.

| DURATION | SET–REP SCHEME | INTENSITY |
|---|---|---|
| WEEKS: 1–4 | 5 × 3 | 90% |
| WEEKS: 5–8 | 5 × 6 | 80% |
| WEEKS: 9–12 | 5 × 12 | 70% |

While little research has been done on this periodization model, one study showed reverse-linear periodization to be inferior for muscle and strength gains when compared to linear periodization (200). However, a study by Rhea and colleagues (201) demonstrated reverse-linear periodization to be more effective than both linear and undulating periodization for eliciting gains in muscular endurance.

# 4.7 NON-LINEAR PERIODIZATION

The difference between the non-linear periodization model and the more traditional models of periodization is that with non-linear periodization the alterations in volume and intensity are made more frequently (197). Rather than training in a certain loading zone for an entire mesocycle, loading zones may vary throughout the mesocycle, or even within the microcycle. An example of three different non-linear periodization protocols is illustrated below.

| WITHIN WEEK | WEEKLY | BI-WEEKLY |
|---|---|---|
| Leg Workout 1: 5 × 5 | Week 1: 5 × 5 | Weeks 1 & 2: 5 × 5 |
| Leg Workout 2: 5 × 15 | Week 2: 5 × 15 | Weeks 3 & 4: 5 × 15 |

As you can see, the alterations in loading zones are made frequently, as opposed to the linear models where changes are made more infrequently. This characteristic of frequent variation may be quite beneficial for strength training, which we touch on later in the chapter.

# 4.8 DAILY UNDULATING PERIODIZATION

Daily undulating periodization is a subset of non-linear periodization, but it is specific to incorporating varied loading zones within the week. This is in contrast to some forms of non-linear periodization, which may vary the loading zones on a weekly or bi-weekly basis (197). Since daily undulating periodization models allow the athlete to train in different loading zones from session to session, this provides a more frequent variation of stimuli than some non-linear models would. Furthermore, the benefit of such frequent alterations in loading zones is that the athlete will maintain the adaptations achieved from training in each loading zone. This is the main criticism of the linear models, as the large amount of time spent in a particular loading zone may cause the athlete to lose the adaptations he or she made from the previous phases (202).

Below is an example of a basic daily undulating periodization model that a lifter wanting to gain size and strength might employ. It must be remembered that substantial variability can exist between daily undulating protocols in regard to the specific loading zones used. For instance, it is not uncommon to use a range from sets of 3 repetitions at the beginning of the week to sets of 20+ repetitions at the end of the week, which was demonstrated in a recent study (203).

| DAY | SET–REP SCHEME | INTENSITY |
|---|---|---|
| MONDAY | $5 \times 3$ | 90% 1RM |
| WEDNESDAY | $5 \times 6$ | 80% 1RM |
| FRIDAY | $5 \times 12$ | 70% 1RM |

## 4.9 BLOCK PERIODIZATION

A more recent periodization model, block periodization incorporates distinct training blocks that are highly concentrated on maximizing a minimal number of target abilities (204–206). There are generally three mesocycle training blocks, each one shorter in duration compared to a traditional linear periodization mesocycle. The purpose of the shorter training blocks is to take advantage of the residual training effect (207), which allows adaptations to be maintained after the cessation of a previous training phase (208). Furthermore, each training block is sequenced in a specific fashion to best prepare the athlete for an upcoming competition. The three blocks (or phases) of the block periodization model consist of the following:

1. **Accumulation**: This phase usually lasts 2–6 weeks and consists of a high volume of work with a low level of intensity. The goal is to build general preparedness, which can include aerobic endurance, muscular strength, and basic coordination (205).
2. **Transmutation**: This is the most exhaustive training block and generally lasts 2–4 weeks. This block reduces training volume and implements more specific training for the given sport (205). This can include a greater emphasis on specific lifts with heavier loading (206).
3. **Realization**: This block can be thought of as a taper period and lasts 1–2 weeks. It is designed to maximize sport-specific skills while allowing sufficient recovery before competition (205). For strength training, volume is kept minimal and an emphasis on specific lifts with very heavy loading is maximized (206).

The completion of all three training blocks represents a "training stage," which is usually followed by a competition. Each training stage generally lasts between 5–10 weeks (205), though they may last slightly longer. This is one of the brighter aspects of block periodization, as it is a viable option for athletes who compete in numerous competitions per year.

# 4.10 THE CONJUGATE SYSTEM

A periodization model that should be reserved for advanced lifters, the conjugate system entails very high workloads that emphasize a particular attribute (e.g., strength) during an "accumulation phase" (usually lasting 4 weeks). This is followed by a "restitution phase" that may last up to 3 weeks (193).

The rationale behind this model is that each accumulation phase is designed for intentional "overreaching" (177), meaning the lifter is pushed to his or her limit of recovery capacity. This can be characterized by expected decrements in training performance. It is at this point that the lifter will move into the restitution phase, which allows for "supercompensation" to occur. It is during this phase that the lifter recovers from the strain of the accumulation phase and is able to come back stronger for the next training cycle.

It should be noted that the restitution phase does not entail complete abstinence from training. On the contrary, the restitution phase allows for a greater emphasis to be shifted toward speed and technique work, while training volume for strength is markedly reduced (177). Therefore, while the accumulation phase places a heavy emphasis on a specific attribute (e.g., strength) with maintenance loads directed to another attribute (e.g., speed), the restitution phase reverses this by prioritizing speed and technique with maintenance loads directed to strength work.

Given the risky nature of this periodization method (it can lead to overtraining if not done correctly), this model should only be reserved for athletes at a very high training status who can tolerate high volume loads (193). Furthermore, the strength and conditioning coach must closely monitor the athlete at all times to ensure that he or she is not being pushed too far during the accumulation phase (193).

# 4.11 AUTOREGULATION

Autoregulation is not so much a strict model of periodization but rather a concept of training. This is because autoregulatory training can be carried out in a number of ways while still accomplishing the same goal. Specifically, autoregulation allows the lifter to continually adjust his or her training based on their rate of progression. This is opposed to strict forms of periodization, which provide specific loading zones to be trained in throughout each training cycle. Autoregulation is far more flexible. Rather than adding weight to the bar in a linear fashion, autoregulation allows the lifter to determine the amount of weight used based on his or her performance for that particular day.

For instance, if lifters are feeling tired and unmotivated to train, they may train with a lighter load than they are regularly accustomed to. Doing this allows the lifter to get his or her volume in while also acting as a form of active recovery. This is more beneficial than having lifters skip a workout or forcing them to lift well beyond what they are capable of at that time.

Given the flexible nature of this training concept, autoregulation can be customized in a variety of ways depending on the lifter's preference. One approach was demonstrated in a study by Mann and colleagues (209), where the researchers compared autoregulatory training to linear periodization in Division 1 football players. Over the 6 week study period, the linear group gradually progressed from high volume and low intensity to low volume and high intensity. The training protocol of the autoregulatory group, on the other hand, was much more elegant.

Essentially, the lifters in the autoregulatory group trained in three different loading zones: three rep max (3RM), six rep max (6RM), and ten rep max (10RM). For each loading zone, the lifters performed 4 sets of exercise. For the sake of simplicity, the researchers used the 6RM loading zone to illustrate the training protocol. The first 3 sets that the lifters performed were based off of their current 6RM. In this case, the lifters performed the first set with 50% of their 6RM weight and the second set with 75% of their 6RM. On the third set, the lifters used 100% of their 6RM for as many repetitions as possible.

The amount of weight used on the fourth set was determined by the result of the third set. So if the lifters performed more than 6 repetitions during their third set, the weight on the fourth set was increased accordingly. This would represent their "new 6RM." The lifter would then perform as many repetitions as possible with the new weight, and the results of that set would determine the amount of weight used for the following week's training.

On the other hand, if the lifter could only perform 6 reps on their third set of exercise, then the weight would remain the same for the fourth set. If the same thing occurred during the fourth set, the weight would stay the same for the following week. Furthermore, if the lifter was unable to complete 6 repetitions with their current weight during the third set, then the weight would be decreased on the fourth set. Again, if the lifter was unable to complete 6 reps on the fourth set, then the weight would be decreased in the following week. An example is illustrated below:

**SET 1:** 10 repetitions @ 50% 6RM

**SET 2:** 6 repetitions @ 75% 6RM

**SET 3:** 100% of 6RM for as many repetitions as possible

**SET 4:** Weight is determined by the result of set 3. The lifter will then perform this new (or unchanged) weight for as many repetitions as possible. The result of this set will determine the weight used for the following week.

As you can see, this system of constant adjustment based on the lifter's progression rate is the core principle of autoregulatory training. It is important to note that this training method can be used for any particular loading zone. Since the researchers in the study felt that a 6RM loading zone was the most beneficial for football players, this was the loading zone that was prioritized. However, if a bodybuilder were to implement autoregulatory training, they may elect a 10RM loading zone and adjust accordingly.

## 4.12 WHICH PERIODIZATION MODEL IS BEST?

Given the variety of periodization models to choose from, it is understandable that a lifter would want to know which one is the most effective. While some studies report no significant differences between the linear and non-linear/undulating models for strength gains (210–217), other studies report an advantage for the non-linear/undulating models (218–224). A meta-analysis by Harries and colleagues (225) found no difference between linear and undulating periodization for eliciting strength gains. Conversely, a more recent meta-analysis (226) found the undulating model to be superior to the linear model for improving maximal strength, with no differences found for power or muscle growth.

Block periodization has shown promise in regard to strength outcomes. Painter and colleagues (227) demonstrated block periodization to produce similar strength increases as daily undulating periodization, even though the block periodization group trained with significantly less volume. While these findings suggest that block periodization may be more efficient for maximizing strength gains, the higher training volume achieved in the daily undulating group may be desirable for bodybuilders looking to maximize hypertrophy (199).

In regard to autoregulation, few studies have compared it to other periodization models. In the study by Mann and colleagues (209), the researchers found that autoregulatory training produced significantly greater strength gains than linear periodization over a 6 week period. While these findings demonstrate potential for this training method, it must be noted that the study was very short in duration, which is a major limitation of periodization research (228).

For the purposes of this book, our training templates will consist of a within-week, non-linear periodization model. This setup will enable the lifter to emphasize both strength and hypertrophy on a frequent basis, as opposed to devoting a singular focus to one over the other for lengthy time periods.

# 5. DIET PRINCIPLES

## 5.1 CALORIES

Calories are a unit of energy (229), and they are the energy our bodies use to sustain life. All of the food we eat comprises macronutrients, and each macronutrient consists of calories. The three primary macronutrients are protein, carbohydrates, and fats. Each macronutrient is made up of a certain amount of calories:

- **Protein**: 4 calories per gram
- **Carbohydrate**: 4 calories per gram
- **Fat**: 9 calories per gram

## 5.2 ENERGY BALANCE

The term "energy balance" refers to the ratio of calories ingested versus calories expended. Since calories are a unit of energy, it is important to understand that any change in bodyweight will be the result of our state of energy balance (230). For instance, to gain weight we must consume more calories than our body burns. This will create a state of "positive energy balance." To lose weight, we must expend more calories than we consume. This results in a state of "negative energy balance" (231). On the other hand, if calorie intake is equal to the amount of calories burned, this will result in neutral energy balance, and no weight change will occur.

This concept of energy balance operates under the first law of thermodynamics, which states that energy can neither be created nor destroyed, but can be transformed from one form to another (229). Therefore, if weight change were to occur irrespective of energy balance, this would essentially violate the laws of physics.

# 5.3 METABOLISM

Metabolism refers to the chemical processes that occur within an organism to sustain life. All of these processes require energy, which can be shown through our metabolic rate. Our metabolic rate can be divided into three categories: resting metabolic rate, active metabolic rate, and diet-induced thermogenesis.

- **Resting metabolic rate:** This refers to the amount of calories our bodies require to operate its organs and nervous system while at rest (232). Therefore, even if we did not perform any physical activity for a period of time, our body would still require calories just to sustain basic functioning. It should be noted that while resting metabolic rate is often used interchangeably with "basal metabolic rate," the measurement practice for the basal rate is slightly different than that of the resting rate. For the sake of simplicity, both terms can be used to assess your calorie needs.

- **Active metabolic rate:** This is the rate that is most variable among individuals (232). This refers to the amount of calories our bodies expend due to physical activity. The higher our degree of physical activity, the more calories our bodies require to sustain that activity. This is why exercise is recommended for weight loss, because it is easier to create a state of negative energy balance when you are expending large amounts of calories throughout the day.

- **Diet-induced thermogenesis:** Also known as the "thermic effect of feeding," this refers to the amount of calories our bodies expend through the absorption and storage of food (232). To put it simply, our body will burn calories every time it consumes calories. This is because the process of digestion requires energy. Generally, diet-induced thermogenesis accounts for roughly 10% of our daily energy output (232). It is also why some foods are better for weight loss than others. While most people believe it is because some foods will not turn into fat while others will, the truth is that some foods are simply more thermogenic than others, meaning they require more energy to be digested than other types of food. There is a general hierarchy of diet-induced thermogenesis when it comes to macronutrients.

## THE HIERARCHY OF DIET-INDUCED THERMOGENESIS

1. **Protein**: This is the most thermogenic macronutrient and has an estimated DIT value of 20–35% (233).

2. **Carbohydrate**: This is the second most thermogenic macronutrient, with an estimated value of 5–15% (233).

3. **Fat**: The thermic effect of fat is a matter of debate, with some authors suggesting a value as low as 0–3% (234) while others suggest it may be equal to carbohydrates (233).

# 5.4 CALCULATING YOUR CALORIE REQUIREMENTS

Given the governance that energy balance has on bodyweight, it is important to know the amount of calories necessary to achieve neutral energy balance. Once we have determined this number, we can adjust it for whether we want to gain or lose weight. It is important to note that too large of a surplus or deficit in energy balance is usually not desirable. In other words, if we take in far more calories than is necessary, we will put on excess body fat, even if we are training hard. Furthermore, if one is looking to lose weight, too much of a calorie deficit may result in muscle and strength impairments (235). This is why it is generally recommended to increase your calorie needs by 10–20% if you are looking to gain weight and to decrease your calorie needs by 10–20% if you are looking to lose weight (236).

A simple method for calculating our resting calorie requirements is presented by the Mifflin-St. Jeor formula (237). According to a review of the most common formulas used to estimate resting calorie requirements, the formula proposed by Mifflin-St. Jeor was shown to be the most accurate (238).

First, we must calculate the values in the Mifflin-St. Jeor formula to determine our resting metabolic rate. Once we have that number, we multiply it by an "activity factor," which is presented in the second chart below. That number will give us our base calorie needs. Once you have that, you can adjust it depending on whether you want to gain weight or lose weight.

## RESTING METABOLIC RATE FORMULA (MIFFLIN-ST. JEOR)

| MEN | (10 × weight in kg) + (6.25 × height in cm) − (5 × age in years) + 5 |
| WOMEN | (10 × weight in kg) + (6.25 × height in cm) − (5 × age in years) − 161 |

Ensure that you calculate the values in each bracket first, then add/subtract each of those values last. Here is an example for how a 30-year-old, 180 cm, 100 kg male would calculate his resting metabolic rate:

**MALE EXAMPLE:** (1000) + (1125) − (150) + 5 = **1980**

For females, the only difference in the formula is the final value. An example of a 30-year-old, 150 cm, 50 kg female is as follows:

**FEMALE EXAMPLE:** (500) + (937.5) − (150) − 161 = **1126.5**

Once you have determined your resting metabolic rate, you will then multiply this value by the activity factor (shown in the next chart) that best suits you. Activity factors are used to account for your active metabolic rate, which is a large determinant of calorie requirements.

## ACTIVITY FACTORS

| ACTIVITY LEVEL | FORMULA |
| --- | --- |
| Sedentary | RMR × 1.2 |
| Lightly Active | RMR × 1.3–1.4 |
| Moderately Active | RMR × 1.5–1.6 |
| Very Active | RMR × 1.7–1.8 |
| Extremely Active | RMR × 1.9–2.2 |

*Values retrieved from Synnott (236).*

Note: Given that most of you will be performing frequent bouts of weight training, your activity level should not be calculated below "Moderately Active". Other factors, such as cardiovascular training and your occupation, will determine whether you should stay in this category or move into the "Very Active" or "Extremely Active" categories.

## ADJUSTING FOR YOUR GOALS

Now that we have determined our base calorie needs to maintain a neutral energy balance, we must adjust it for whether we are looking to gain weight or lose weight. In both cases, 10–20% of our calorie needs is a good amount to aim for (236). By adding or subtracting this value from our base calorie requirements, we can expect to gain muscle or lose fat at a moderate pace that will not disturb our body composition via excessive fat gain or muscle loss.

# 5.5 PROTEIN

Protein is the most essential macronutrient for muscle growth. It is composed of amino acids, which are the building blocks of muscle tissue. The amino acid leucine is of particular importance, given its potency at stimulating muscle protein synthesis (239–246). Interestingly, higher protein intakes have also been associated with greater strength gains compared to lower intakes (247).

Not only is an optimal protein intake mandatory for maximizing muscle and strength gains, it can also provide benefits for those looking to lose fat. First, protein is the most thermogenic macronutrient (248). Second, protein is the most satiating macronutrient (249, 250). In other words, protein has a pronounced effect on making us feel full after food consumption. This is why high-protein diets are very effective for those looking to lose weight, as their effect on satiety makes it easier to consume fewer calories throughout the day. Furthermore, a high protein intake is crucial for anyone aiming to retain muscle mass while in a caloric deficit (251–258).

## RECOMMENDED INTAKE

When at neutral energy balance or in a caloric surplus, an intake of ~2 grams of protein per kilogram of bodyweight has been recommended for strength training (259). When in a caloric deficit, a range of 1.8–2.7 grams of protein per kilogram of bodyweight has been proposed to prevent muscle loss while dieting (260). Other experts have suggested that a range of 2.3–3.1 grams of protein per kilogram of *fat-free mass* may be the most protective against muscle loss during calorie restriction (261).

It must be stressed, however, that to *maximize* muscle growth a caloric surplus is necessary. In fact, experts have stated that calorie intake may be more important than protein intake for promoting muscle gains (262).

# 5.6 CARBOHYDRATES

Carbohydrates are an excellent energy source for our bodies. When ingested, carbohydrates can be stored in our muscles and liver as glycogen (263). This is of great importance for athletes, as muscle glycogen acts as an energy reserve that can be used during bouts of intense physical activity. In regard to strength training, some studies have shown carbohydrate restriction to have a negative effect on training performance (264, 265), whereas others have not (266, 267).

## RECOMMENDED INTAKE

For strength athletes, Slater and Phillips (268) recommend a range of 4–7 grams of carbohydrates per kilogram of bodyweight. It must be stressed, however, that it is completely up to the individual on how many carbs they prefer to keep in their diet. While some lifters prefer a lot of carbs to perform optimally, others prefer low-carb dieting. As long as your carb intake does not interfere with your ability to maintain an optimal protein intake, then your carb requirements can be determined based on preference.

## CARBOHYDRATES AND FAT LOSS

Certainly one of the biggest dietary myths is the notion that carbohydrates are inherently fattening. This generally results in fitness gurus preaching the importance of eliminating carbs from your diet to induce fat loss. Interestingly, the majority of evidence does not support these claims. Specifically, when calories are matched between groups, the amount of carbohydrates consumed has no impact on weight gain or weight loss (269–279).

While it is generally agreed that carbohydrates will not make you fat if calories are controlled, there is merit to restricting them if you are trying to lose weight. First, by restricting carbs you are also restricting yourself of an array of food choices. This will make it less tempting to overconsume calories (280).

Second, restricting carbs generally forces you to increase your protein intake to make up for the lack of carbs. Since we already discussed the effect that protein can have on fat loss via satiety, it is understandable that most people who go on low-carb diets report weight loss. Unfortunately, many of these individuals blame carbs as the culprit for their initial weight gain, when in reality it was the result of a prolonged positive energy balance.

## RECOMMENDATIONS FOR FAT LOSS

Given these findings, if you are trying to lose body fat, you should emphasize maintaining a caloric deficit with a high protein intake. While restricting carbs may make it easier for some individuals to adhere to these principles, others who enjoy carbs can maintain them in their diet as long as they do not create a caloric surplus.

# 5.7 FATS

Fat is a critical macronutrient for bodily functioning. Specific to athletes, dietary fat is crucial for maintaining healthy androgen levels; numerous studies have shown fat intake to have a significant effect on testosterone production (281–285).

## TESTOSTERONE AND BODY COMPOSITION

It is undeniable that testosterone levels beyond the "natural" range can induce profound muscle growth (286–290). However, whether testosterone levels within the natural range can impact muscle growth is less clear. Interestingly, a recent study (291) demonstrated that men in the highest quartiles for testosterone had more muscle and less body fat than men in the bottom quartile. While these findings provide intriguing insights into the impact of natural testosterone levels and body composition, it is important to note that these results show a correlational relationship, which does not infer causation (292).

## RECOMMENDED INTAKE

While fat intake can vary depending on the person, a general recommendation provided by Lambert and colleagues (293) is that about 15–20% of your total calories should come from fat to maintain healthy androgen levels.

## 5.8 MEAL FREQUENCY

### MEAL FREQUENCY AND WEIGHT LOSS

Another common misconception regarding optimal eating habits is the effect of meal frequency on body composition. While many people preach the importance of eating numerous meals throughout the day to "boost metabolism," this notion has been refuted in research (294–298). Furthermore, numerous studies have shown meal frequency to be irrelevant for weight loss under calorie-controlled conditions (299–302).

### MEAL FREQUENCY AND MUSCLE MASS

While it appears conclusive that meal frequency is irrelevant for weight loss, whether it has an impact on muscle retention (or growth) is highly controversial. While some studies show a benefit of higher meal frequencies for muscle retention (303–305), others do not (306, 307).

A meta-analysis by Schoenfeld and colleagues (308) initially revealed a benefit of higher meal frequencies for muscle mass. However, sensitivity analysis revealed that these findings were highly influenced by the results of one study (305), and that removal of this study negated the influence of meal frequency on muscle mass.

Research on the effect of protein distribution has also been controversial. Mamerow and colleagues (309) demonstrated that an even protein distribution (three servings of ~30 grams) was more effective at stimulating 24 hour protein synthesis rates versus a bolus approach (~10 g, 15 g, 65 g). Supporting these findings is a study by Arnal and colleagues (310), which compared the effects of a spread protein intake versus a bolus approach in young women. While not deemed statistically significant, the spread intake resulted in 1.5 times greater nitrogen retention than the bolus approach. Conversely, multiple studies have demonstrated no advantage of a spread protein distribution on protein balance or muscle mass compared to a bolus approach (311–314).

A study by Areta and colleagues (315) demonstrated that a moderate distribution of protein (four servings of 20 grams protein) was superior to two protein servings (2 × 40 grams protein) and 8 protein servings (8 x 10 grams protein) for stimulating protein synthesis. While this study provides additional insight into the matter of meal frequency and muscle growth, the choice of study design makes it difficult to extrapolate these results to real-world eating habits (316).

## RECOMMENDATIONS

Given the evidence to date, there appears to be no optimal meal frequency for promoting weight loss, which is contrary to what the mainstream media continues to preach to the public. In regard to muscle growth, the answer is less clear. Some experts advocate a spread pattern of 3–4 meals per day (260); however, this recommendation remains controversial given the current evidence (308). Furthermore, most studies on meal frequency do not include resistance training, therefore making it difficult to extrapolate their results to a strength training population. Given the conflicting findings in the research, it should be left up to personal preference on how many meals per day you consume.

# 5.9 MEAL TIMING

Another controversial aspect of nutrition for strength training is the role that meal timing plays on muscle growth. Specifically, this refers to the idea that there is a short "anabolic window of opportunity" around a training session where protein must be ingested to induce muscle growth. While many experts have bought into this notion (317–319), the research on the topic has been greatly divided. Multiple studies have shown a benefit to timing protein consumption close to a training session (320, 321), whereas others have not (322–325).

To gain some clarity on the topic, a meta-analysis by Schoenfeld and colleagues (326) sought to determine whether timing protein ingestion in close proximity to training had an effect on muscle growth. After analysis of the data, the researchers found a beneficial effect of protein timing on hypertrophy, but not on strength. However, once the researchers controlled for total protein intake, there was no significant effect of protein timing on muscle growth. These results suggest that total protein intake per day is the overriding factor to promote muscle growth, and that protein timing appears to have a negligible effect.

## RECOMMENDATIONS

Given these findings, it is apparent that total daily protein intake should be prioritized ahead of protein timing. In regard to when protein should be consumed, that can be left to your discretion. Having said that, there is certainly no harm in ingesting protein around training, and it is still encouraged if not deemed inconvenient by the individual. This is especially true for physique competitors where any tiny benefit can mean the difference between winning and losing a competition.

It should also be mentioned that individuals who engage in fasted training would benefit from immediate post-workout protein consumption. This is because muscle breakdown rates are heightened in a fasted state (327), thereby necessitating the need for immediate protein consumption following training (328).

## 5.10 POST-WORKOUT NUTRITION

### PROTEIN DOSE

Another frequently asked question in fitness circles is what the optimal amount of protein dose is to maximize protein synthesis post-workout. This usually garners a range of responses, usually lying between 20–30 grams. This response is in line with what most experts suggest, as 20–25 grams of protein post-workout appears sufficient to maximize protein synthesis (329).

Having said this, recent evidence suggests that the optimal protein dose post-workout may be dependent on the amount of muscle groups worked. In other words, someone who performed a full-body workout may require more than this 25 gram threshold to maximize protein synthesis versus someone who only trained one or two muscle groups. This was demonstrated in a study by Macnaughton and colleagues (330), where the researchers found that 40 grams of protein stimulated protein synthesis to a greater degree than 20 grams of protein following a full-body training session.

Furthermore, it should be noted that age may also play an important role in the amount of protein needed to maximize protein synthesis post-workout. This is because older individuals are less sensitive to protein consumption than younger individuals (331), thereby necessitating the need for higher protein intakes (at least 40 grams) following training (332).

### CARBOHYDRATE INTAKE

While it has been suggested that carbohydrate intake following training can help to inhibit muscle protein breakdown (333), this is only true if your protein intake post-workout is unreasonably small. This was shown in a study by Staples and colleagues (334), which demonstrated that when an adequate amount of protein is ingested following training, additional carbs do not provide an additive effect for inhibiting muscle protein breakdown.

## RECOMMENDATIONS

Given the evidence, it is clear that as long as an adequate protein dose is consumed following training, then consuming carbohydrates will have no further effect on promoting a hypertrophic response. Having said that, there is certainly no drawback to consuming carbs post-workout—if anything, it would allow the body to quickly replenish muscle glycogen stores (335) that will be partially depleted from training (336).

In regard to protein intake following training, the optimal dose appears to depend on different factors, including age and the amount of muscles trained in a session. Younger lifters who train singular body parts will be fine consuming 20–25 grams of protein post-workout, whereas older lifters should consume a minimum of 40 grams of protein following training. Furthermore, when many muscle groups are trained in a session (such as a full-body routine), a minimum of 40 grams of protein may be necessary to maximize protein synthesis, regardless of the lifter's age.

# 5.11 HYDRATION

While its importance is often overlooked, staying properly hydrated plays a pivotal role in the ability for your muscles to work at maximum capacity. This was demonstrated in two studies (337, 338), which showed that dehydration significantly impaired weight-training performance in male subjects.

## WATER REQUIREMENTS

It is important to understand that recommending a base level of water intake to the general population will never be completely accurate. This is because water requirements can vary widely between individuals and are influenced by factors such as body size and activity level. Fortunately, Popkin and colleagues (339) presented a table of estimated water requirements that correspond with calorie requirements.

Based on an average of these estimates for both male and female adults, the requirement for adequate water intake would roughly equate to 1.4 milliliters of water per calorie of food intake.

# 6. INTERMITTENT FASTING

# 6.1 OVERVIEW OF INTERMITTENT FASTING

Intermittent fasting has emerged as a popular trend for fat loss. Generally speaking, the goal of most intermittent fasting regimens is to reduce calorie intake through incorporating routine fasts throughout the day or week, followed by designated feeding periods. Generally, there are four forms of intermittent fasting (340):

1. **Time-restricted feeding**: Consists of eating a day's worth of calories in a condensed feeding window (generally 4–8 hours). Most time-restricted feeding programs allocate the feeding period to the afternoon or evening.

2. **Ramadan fasting:** This form of intermittent fasting is essentially time-restricted feeding done for religious reasons rather than improving body composition. It should be noted that Ramadan fasting typically incorporates fluid restriction during the fasting period, whereas other forms of intermittent fasting do not.

3. **Whole-day fasting:** Consists of one or two daily fasts per week where a minimal amount of calories are consumed during the "fasting days," with ad libitum (unrestricted) calorie consumption during the remaining days. This method has shown promise as an alternative weight loss strategy to daily calorie restriction (341, 342).

4. **Alternate-day fasting:** Consists of daily alternations between ad libitum calorie intake and very little calorie intake. This method has also shown promise for reducing fat mass (343) and preserving muscle mass (344).

# 6.2 INTERMITTENT FASTING AND MUSCLE GROWTH

There has been a great deal of controversy surrounding intermittent fasting's effect on muscle growth. The common assumption is that going for long periods of time without eating cannot be good for muscle tissue, and thus practicing intermittent fasting may impede one's ability to maximize muscle growth. So far, this notion remains highly questionable, as demonstrated in the section on meal frequency. The problem with meal frequency studies, however, is that almost none of them include resistance training. To date, only a few studies that have compared intermittent fasting to a traditional eating schedule have incorporated resistance training into the design. We review the most recent ones below.

## 20 HOUR FASTING VERSUS REGULAR EATING

A study by Tinsley and colleagues (345) compared a regular eating group to a time-restricted feeding group while participating in an 8 week weight-training program. The regular eating group was permitted to eat normally throughout the day, while the time-restricted feeding group consumed all of their calories within a 4 hour feeding window 4 days per week. The remaining 3 days were training days, where both groups were allowed to eat regularly throughout the day.

At the end of the study period, the regular eating group gained more muscle than the time-restricted feeding group, although the time-restricted feeding group had greater strength improvements than the regular eating group. While these findings are quite compelling, it should be noted that certain variables in the study were not controlled for. One of which was protein intake, as it was reported that the regular eating group consumed 1.4 grams of protein per kilogram of bodyweight whereas the time-restricted feeding group only consumed 1 gram per kilogram of bodyweight. Furthermore, training sessions were not supervised, which is another limitation acknowledged by the researchers.

## 16 HOUR FASTING VERSUS REGULAR EATING

Moro and colleagues (346) conducted another study on time-restricted feeding, this one comparing the effects of a 16 hour daily fast to a regular eating pattern during an 8 week weight-training program. Meal frequency between groups was identical (three meals per day), with the only difference being that the fasting group consumed their meals between 1 p.m. and 9 p.m. whereas the regular eating group consumed their meals between 8 a.m. and 9 p.m. Weight training was carried out in a supervised fashion 3 days per week. Contrary to the first study, protein was matched between groups and was of an optimal amount for strength-training standards. At the end of the study period, there were no differences between the two groups for muscle or strength gains.

While these findings are quite compelling, it should be noted that in both studies the intermittent fasting groups did not train in a fasted state, which is a common practice for many intermittent fasting practitioners. Whether this would have influenced the results is unclear, but research on Ramadan fasting has shown no disadvantage of fasted weight training for muscle growth (347).

## CONCLUSIONS

Given the current evidence, intermittent fasting does not appear to detrimentally affect strength gains compared to regular eating. In regard to muscle growth, the evidence is less clear. Given Schoenfeld's meta-analysis on meal frequency (308), as well as the tighter control of Moro's study (346), it is reasonable to assume that if intermittent fasting does have any impact on muscle growth it is likely minimal at best. Further studies are needed to draw firmer conclusions on this topic.

# 7. SUPPLEMENTS

# 7.1 CREATINE MONOHYDRATE

Undoubtedly the most effective training supplement on the market (348), creatine monohydrate has been proven for decades to be highly effective for enhancing strength gains (349–366). To illustrate its potency, Jówko and colleagues (367) demonstrated that creatine supplementation resulted in a near threefold greater increase in accumulative strength gains compared to a placebo.

## HOW IT WORKS

It is suggested that creatine increases the availability of ATP (adenosine triphosphate) to the muscles during exercise (368), thus allowing them to work harder and longer. In effect, this produces significant increases in training performance (369), which may positively affect hypertrophy outcomes on top of strength gains. Furthermore, a study by Parise and colleagues (370) demonstrated that creatine ingestion reduced leucine oxidation in men. This finding suggests that in addition to increasing strength performance, creatine may also provide an anti-catabolic effect.

## WHEN TO TAKE CREATINE

A common question among lifters is whether it is better to ingest creatine prior to training or immediately after training. While there has not been much research on the topic, one study (371) demonstrated superior gains in strength and body composition in the group that ingested creatine post-workout versus pre-workout. It should be noted, however, that the study duration was quite short (4 weeks).

## SAFETY OF CREATINE USE

Another common concern surrounding creatine usage relates to its safety. While there is speculation that long-term creatine usage may pose certain health risks, this has not been supported by research. For instance, Kreider and colleagues (372) examined the effects of 21 months of creatine consumption in college football players. At the end of the study, no adverse effects on health markers were observed. These findings are in accordance with multiple review papers on the topic (373–376), all of which conclude that there is no valid evidence to suggest that creatine adversely affects health status in healthy individuals. In fact, recent research has suggested that creatine may even provide neuroprotective benefits (377). While these findings suggest that creatine usage presents no health risks, regular medical checkups would still be wise during prolonged creatine supplementation.

## 7.2 WHEY PROTEIN

Whey protein powder is an excellent solution for individuals who cannot meet their protein requirements from food alone. This is generally the case for people adhering to weight-loss diets, as protein requirements may increase during periods of calorie restriction (378). Considering most whey powders provide high doses of protein at low calorie servings, this presents another attractive feature of protein supplementation to lifters aiming to lose body fat while retaining muscle mass. Furthermore, whey protein is regarded as a high-quality protein source (379, 380), especially given its high leucine content (381).

## 7.3 BRANCHED-CHAIN AMINO ACIDS

A popular supplement among bodybuilders (38), branched-chain amino acids (BCAAs) are commonly used to stimulate protein synthesis and minimize protein degradation in an effort to enhance muscle growth. Despite their popularity, evidence for the long-term effectiveness of BCAA supplementation has been controversial. Many studies have shown BCAAs to reduce muscle soreness from training (382–385), though these findings are not universal (386). A published abstract by Stoppani and colleagues (387) reported that BCAA supplementation improved muscle and strength gains to a significantly greater extent than both whey protein and carbohydrates over an 8 week training period. Supporting these findings, Dudgeon and colleagues (388) demonstrated that BCAA supplementation retained muscle mass and increased strength to a greater extent than carbohydrates during an 8 week, calorie-restricted training program. It should be noted, however, that the results from this study have been criticized because of discrepancies found in the reported data (389).

Contrasting these findings, Spillane and colleagues (390) showed that BCAAs had no positive effect on muscle or strength gains over an 8 week training period. Furthermore, Churchward-Venne and colleagues (245) demonstrated that a BCAA blend was no more effective than leucine at stimulating protein synthesis. It is suggested that this is due to an antagonistic effect between BCAAs, since they compete for absorption (391).

Given these conflicting reports, BCAA supplementation should be left up to the individual until further research can draw more definitive conclusions. From a theoretical standpoint, lifters who engage in fasted training might benefit from supplementing with BCAAs before or during exercise to improve muscle protein balance. However, given the results of Churchward-Venne's study (245), leucine alone may be more effective.

## 7.4 GLUTAMINE

Many strength athletes consume glutamine under the assumption that it will aid in muscle recovery and thereby promote superior adaptations from training. This is logical given that research has suggested glutamine to have anti-catabolic effects on muscle tissue (392). Unfortunately, this notion has not been supported by research, as a 6 week training study (393) failed to show a beneficial effect of glutamine supplementation on muscle or strength gains in young adults. While it appears at present that glutamine supplementation is unwarranted for enhancing muscle and strength gains, longer-term trials are needed to determine if this is the case.

## 7.5 CAFFEINE

Despite its prevalent use among bodybuilders (394), the effectiveness of caffeine for improving strength performance is unclear. In a recent meta-analysis (395), caffeine ingestion appeared to have no effect on strength, but it did provide a benefit for muscular endurance. Given these findings, it is possible that caffeine may be beneficial during high-repetition training, which may aid in increasing training volume.

## 7.6 BETA-ALANINE

An emerging supplement in the strength-training community, beta-alanine is used to increase muscle carnosine concentrations (396), which may improve work capacity (397). This notion has been supported in multiple meta-analyses (398, 399), which demonstrated that beta-alanine supplementation significantly increased exercise capacity compared to a placebo. In regard to strength training, the research has generally been favorable. Multiple studies have shown beta-alanine to be effective for increasing training volume (400, 401), which would theoretically enhance muscle gains over the long term. These results have led experts to suggest that the benefits of beta-alanine are strongest when training in high repetition ranges (402). It should be noted, however, that little is known about the long-term safety of beta-alanine supplementation (394). While it appears to be relatively safe over the short term (403), further research is needed to determine any negative health effects from long-term usage.

# 8. TRAINING TEMPLATES

## 8.1 UNTRAINED

*WEEKS 1–7*

### DAY 1: LEGS [STRENGTH]

Barbell Squats 4 × 6
Leg Curls 3 × 6

### DAY 2: CHEST & SHOULDERS [STRENGTH]

Bench Press 4 × 6
Shoulder Press 3 × 5

### DAY 3: LEGS & BACK [STRENGTH]

Deadlifts 4 × 6
One-arm Dumbbell Rows 3 × 5

### DAY 4: OFF

### DAY 5: LEGS [HYPERTROPHY]

Barbell Squats 4 × 10
Leg Curls 3 × 10

### DAY 6: CHEST & SHOULDERS [HYPERTROPHY]

Bench Press 4 × 10
Shoulder Press 3 × 10

### DAY 7: BACK [HYPERTROPHY]

Pull-ups 4 × 10 (or failure)

Barbell Rows 3 × 10

## DAY 8: OFF

## *WEEK 8: UNLOADING CYCLE*

## DAY 1: LEGS [STRENGTH]

Barbell Squats 2 × 6
Leg Curls 1 × 6

## DAY 2: CHEST & SHOULDERS [STRENGTH]

Bench Press 2 × 6
Shoulder Press 1 × 5

## DAY 3: LEGS & BACK [STRENGTH]

Deadlifts 2 × 6
One-arm Dumbbell Rows 1 × 6

## DAY 4: OFF

## DAY 5: LEGS [HYPERTROPHY]

Barbell Squats 2 × 10
Leg Curls 1 × 10

## DAY 6: CHEST & SHOULDERS [HYPERTROPHY]

Bench Press 2 × 10
Shoulder Press 1 × 10

## DAY 7: BACK [HYPERTROPHY]

Pull-ups 2 × 10 (or failure)
Barbell Rows 1 × 10

## DAY 8: OFF

## 8.2 RECREATIONALLY TRAINED

### *WEEK 1*

### DAY 1: LEGS [STRENGTH]

Barbell Squats 6 × 3
Leg Curls 3 × 6

### DAY 2: CHEST & SHOULDERS [STRENGTH]

Bench Press 6 × 3
Weighted Dips 3 × 5
Shoulder Press 3 × 5

### DAY 3: LEGS & BACK [STRENGTH]

Deadlifts 6 × 3
Weighted Pull-ups 3 × 5

### DAY 4: OFF

### DAY 5: LEGS [HYPERTROPHY]

Barbell Squats 6 × 10
Leg Curls 3 × 10

### DAY 6: CHEST & SHOULDERS [HYPERTROPHY]

Bench Press 6 × 10
Incline Bench Press 3 × 10
Shoulder Press 3 × 10

### DAY 7: BACK [HYPERTROPHY]

Pull-ups 6 × 10
Barbell Rows 3 × 10

**DAY 8: OFF**

*WEEK 2*

**DAY 1: LEGS [STRENGTH]**

Barbell Squats 6 × 3
Leg Curls 3 × 6

**DAY 2: CHEST & SHOULDERS [STRENGTH]**

Bench Press 6 × 3
Weighted Dips 3 × 5
Shoulder Press 3 × 5

**DAY 3: LEGS & BACK [STRENGTH]**

Deadlifts 6 × 3
Weighted Pull-ups 3 × 5

**DAY 4: OFF**

**DAY 5: LEGS [HYPERTROPHY]**

Barbell Squats 3 × 20
Leg Curls 2 × 20

**DAY 6: CHEST & SHOULDERS [HYPERTROPHY]**

Bench Press 3 × 20
Incline Bench Press 2 × 20

Shoulder Press 2 × 20

## DAY 7: BACK [HYPERTROPHY]

Pull-ups 3 × 20 (or failure)
Barbell Rows 2 × 20

## DAY 8: OFF

*WEEK 3*

## DAY 1: LEGS [STRENGTH]

Barbell Squats 6 × 3
Leg Curls 3 × 6

## DAY 2: CHEST & SHOULDERS [STRENGTH]

Bench Press 6 × 3
Weighted Dips 3 × 5
Shoulder Press 3 × 5

## DAY 3: LEGS & BACK [STRENGTH]

Deadlifts 6 × 3
Weighted Pull-ups 3 × 5

## DAY 4: OFF

## DAY 5: LEGS [HYPERTROPHY]

Barbell Squats 6 × 10
Leg Curls 3 × 10

## DAY 6: CHEST & SHOULDERS [HYPERTROPHY]

Bench Press 6 × 10
Incline Bench Press 3 × 10
Shoulder Press 3 × 10

## DAY 7: BACK [HYPERTROPHY]

Pull-ups 6 × 10
Barbell Rows 3 × 10

## DAY 8: OFF

## *WEEK 4: UNLOADING CYCLE*

## DAY 1: LEGS [STRENGTH]

Barbell Squats 3 × 3
Leg Curls 1 × 6

## DAY 2: CHEST & SHOULDERS [STRENGTH]

Bench Press 3 × 3
Weighted Dips 1 × 5
Shoulder Press 1 × 5

## DAY 3: LEGS & BACK [STRENGTH]

Deadlifts 3 × 3
Weighted Pull-ups 1 × 5

## DAY 4: OFF

## DAY 5: LEGS [HYPERTROPHY]

Barbell Squats 1 × 20
Leg Curls 1 × 20

## DAY 6: CHEST & SHOULDERS [HYPERTROPHY]

Bench Press 1 × 20
Incline Bench Press 1 × 20
Shoulder Press 1 × 20

## DAY 7: BACK [HYPERTROPHY]

Pull-ups 3 × 10
Barbell Rows 1 × 20

## DAY 8: OFF

## 8.3 HIGHLY TRAINED

### *WEEK 1: BASELINE VOLUME*

### DAY 1: LEGS [STRENGTH]

Barbell Squats 6 × 3
Leg Curls 3 × 6

### DAY 2: CHEST & SHOULDERS [STRENGTH]

Bench Press 6 × 3
Weighted Dips 3 × 5
Shoulder Press 3 × 5

### DAY 3: LEGS & BACK [STRENGTH]

Deadlifts 6 × 3
Weighted Pull-ups 3 × 5

### DAY 4: OFF

### DAY 5: LEGS [HYPERTROPHY]

Barbell Squats 6 × 10
Leg Curls 3 × 10

### DAY 6: CHEST & SHOULDERS [HYPERTROPHY]

Bench Press 6 × 10
Incline Bench Press 3 × 10
Shoulder Press 3 × 10

### DAY 7: BACK [HYPERTROPHY]

Pull-ups 6 × 10
Barbell Rows 3 × 10

**DAY 8: OFF**

***WEEK 2: VOLUME RAMP 1***

**DAY 1: LEGS [STRENGTH]**

Barbell Squats 8 × 3
Leg Curls 3 × 6

**DAY 2: CHEST & SHOULDERS [STRENGTH]**

Bench Press 8 × 3
Weighted Dips 3 × 5
Shoulder Press 3 × 5

**DAY 3: LEGS & BACK [STRENGTH]**

Deadlifts 8 × 3
Weighted Pull-ups 3 × 5

**DAY 4: OFF**

**DAY 5: LEGS [HYPERTROPHY]**

Barbell Squats 4 × 20
Leg Curls 2 × 20

**DAY 6: CHEST & SHOULDERS [HYPERTROPHY]**

Bench Press 4 × 20
Incline Bench Press 2 × 20

Shoulder Press 2 × 20

## DAY 7: BACK [HYPERTROPHY]

Pull-ups 4 × 20 (or failure)
Barbell Rows 2 × 20

## DAY 8: OFF

### *WEEK 3: VOLUME RAMP 2*

## DAY 1: LEGS [STRENGTH]

Barbell Squats 10 × 3
Leg Curls 3 × 6

## DAY 2: CHEST & SHOULDERS [STRENGTH]

Bench Press 10 × 3
Weighted Dips 3 × 5
Shoulder Press 3 × 5

## DAY 3: LEGS & BACK [STRENGTH]

Deadlifts 10 × 3
Weighted Pull-ups 3 × 5

## DAY 4: OFF

## DAY 5: LEGS [HYPERTROPHY]

Barbell Squats 10 × 10
Leg Curls 4 × 10

## DAY 6: CHEST & SHOULDERS [HYPERTROPHY]

Bench Press 10 × 10
Incline Bench Press 4 × 10
Shoulder Press 4 × 10

## DAY 7: BACK [HYPERTROPHY]

Pull-ups 10 × 10
Barbell Rows 4 × 10

## DAY 8: OFF

*WEEK 4: UNLOADING CYCLE*

## DAY 1: LEGS [STRENGTH]

Barbell Squats 3 × 3
Leg Curls 1 × 6

## DAY 2: CHEST & SHOULDERS [STRENGTH]

Bench Press 3 × 3
Weighted Dips 1 × 5
Shoulder Press 1 × 5

## DAY 3: LEGS & BACK [STRENGTH]

Deadlifts 3 × 3
Weighted Pull-ups 1 × 5

## DAY 4: OFF

## DAY 5: LEGS [HYPERTROPHY]

Barbell Squats 2 × 20
Leg Curls 1 × 20

## DAY 6: CHEST & SHOULDERS [HYPERTROPHY]

Bench Press 2 × 20
Incline Bench Press 1 × 20
Shoulder Press 1 × 10

## DAY 7: BACK [HYPERTROPHY]

Pull-ups 3 × 10
Barbell Rows 1 × 20

## DAY 8: OFF

## 8.4 LOADING RECOMMENDATIONS

| REPETITIONS PER SET | % 1RM |
|---|---|
| 3 | 85 |
| 5 | 80–85 |
| 6 | 80 |
| 10 | 65–75 |
| 20 | 50–55 |

## 8.5 CATEGORY RECOMMENDATIONS

| TRAINING STATUS | YEARS OF EXPERIENCE |
|---|---|
| Untrained | 0–1 |
| Recreationally Trained | 1–5 |
| Highly Trained | 5+ |

**NOTE**: The categories provided are based on recommendations proposed by Rhea (404). It is important to note that "training experience" refers to your years spent consistently training without long breaks. Furthermore, it must be stressed that the above recommendations are estimates and that variability may exist between individuals in regard to training tolerance. Therefore, it is important that you use your discretion to assess which training template is best suited for your current fitness level.

## 8.6 NOTES ON THE PROGRAMS

As you can see, the training templates provided consist of "strength" days at the beginning of the week followed by "hypertrophy" days near the end of the week. While substantial muscle growth can occur when training with low repetitions during the strength days, the higher volume of the hypertrophy days will preferentially enhance muscle growth.

During the hypertrophy days (following the "Untrained" template), it is recommended to alternate (weekly) between sets of 10 and sets of 20 repetitions to maximally stimulate each muscle fiber type. In other words, while training in lower repetition ranges may preferentially stimulate the type II muscle fibers, the longer time under tension provided from the sets of 20 repetitions may preferentially target your type I fibers.

It should also be understood that these routines are templates and not strict programs. Therefore, while the routines emphasize compound movements, additional isolation exercises can be incorporated based on your preferences. If you elect to do so, including leg curls into your leg days (as shown in the templates) may be wise, as these have been shown to produce a high level of hamstring activation (405).

Furthermore, while the usefulness of performing isolation exercises alongside compound exercises has been questioned (406, 407), isolation movements can still be incorporated to correct muscle imbalances (i.e., "weak points") in the individual (408).

# CLOSING STATEMENTS

As you can see, there have been decades of research on the best training and dietary practices for maximizing muscle and strength development. While adhering to a basic training routine that emphasizes progressive overload will take you far, if your goal is to reach your maximum potential then more intricate strategies will be necessary. The purpose of this book is to provide you with a detailed description of these strategies in hopes that they will aid you in reaching your fullest potential.

Good luck.

# GLOSSARY

**1RM** – Stands for "one repetition maximum." This means the maximum amount of weight you can lift for one repetition.

**AD LIBITUM** – A Latin term meaning "at one's pleasure." In dietary studies, this term is generally used to indicate unrestricted food intake.

**ANABOLIC** – Growth of a bodily tissue.

**ANABOLISM** – The anabolic process.

**AMINO ACID** – A building block of proteins.

**ANDROGEN** – A steroid hormone responsible for male characteristics. Testosterone is an example of an androgen.

**ATP** – Stands for adenosine triphosphate. Refers to the energy currency of a cell.

**BODY COMPOSITION** – The amount of fat and muscle mass on the body. Improving body composition usually refers to maximizing muscle mass and minimizing body fat.

**CALORIE** – A unit of energy that is required by the body to sustain life.

**CATABOLIC** – The breaking down of molecules into smaller units. A catabolic state is required for muscle loss.

**COGNITION** – Mental processes in the brain.

**COMPOUND EXERCISE** – A multi-joint movement. These are generally considered the most effective types of exercises for producing muscle and strength gains.

**CONCENTRIC ACTION** – The shortening of a muscle. An example would be the upward phase of a biceps curl.

**CONCURRENT TRAINING** – Pairing resistance training and aerobic training within a training regimen.

**DOSE-RESPONSE RELATIONSHIP** – The effect on an organism that is dependent on the dosage of a stressor. For instance, the degree of muscle growth may be dependent on the dosage of training volume (up to a point).

**ECCENTRIC ACTION** – The lengthening of a muscle. An example would be the downward phase of a biceps curl.

**EFFECT SIZE** – A statistical measurement used to determine the magnitude of a treatment effect.

**ENERGY BALANCE** – The ratio of calories consumed versus calories expended.

**EXERCISE CAPACITY** – The ability to sustain maximal physical exertion.

**FAT-FREE MASS** – Refers to bodyweight that does not include fat mass.

**GLYCOGEN** – Stored carbohydrates within the muscle and liver.

**GROWTH HORMONE** – A peptide hormone considered to have anabolic and catabolic properties.

**HYPERTROPHY** – The enlargement of organs or tissue caused by an increase in its cell size.

**INTENSITY** – Generally refers to the amount of weight lifted. Is usually determined from a 1RM percentage.

**INTERMITTENT FASTING** – Consists of the abstinence (or marked reduction) of food consumption for regular time periods.

**ISOLATION EXERCISE** – A single-joint movement.

**LEUCINE** – An essential amino acid that regulates protein synthesis.

**LOAD** – Refers to weight (mass).

**LOADING ZONE** – Can refer to a repetition range.

**MAXIMAL STRENGTH** – The maximal amount of force that can be generated for a single repetition.

**MACRONUTRIENT** – A substance that provides energy. The three primary macronutrients are protein, carbohydrates, and fats.

**META-ANALYSIS** – A combination of data from multiple studies.

**METABOLIC STRESS** – Consists of the accumulation of metabolites as a result of resistance training. Metabolic stress is suggested to be a determinant of muscle growth.

**METABOLISM** – The chemical processes that occur in an organism to sustain life.

**MOTOR UNIT** – A unit made up of a motor neuron and muscle fibers. These are used to promote muscle contractions.

**MUSCLE GLYCOGEN** – Stored carbohydrates within the muscle that is used as an energy source during intensive physical activity.

**MUSCLE HYPERTROPHY** – The enlargement of a muscle.

**MUSCULAR ENDURANCE** – The ability of a muscle (or group of muscles) to sustain repeated contractions without tiring.

**NEGATIVE ENERGY BALANCE** – When the amount of calories expended exceeds the amount of calories consumed. This is required for weight loss.

**NEURAL** – Relates to the nervous system.

**NEUROPROTECTIVE** – Protection against neuronal damage/dysfunction as the result of acute trauma or neurodegenerative diseases.

**NITROGEN** – A key element of an amino acid.

**NITROGEN BALANCE** – Refers to nitrogen intake versus nitrogen loss. This is commonly used in studies to measure protein retention.

**OVERREACHING** – Intentionally training to a point where the stress exceeds the body's ability to recover. These periods are used to create a "rebound effect" following recovery from training. This can result in the body becoming significantly stronger following the recovery period.

**PERIODIZATION** – A cyclic structure of training designed to maximize performance, manage fatigue, and minimize plateaus.

**PLACEBO** – A substance that has no therapeutic effect. These are used in experiments to trick the placebo group into thinking they are receiving the actual treatment drug.

**PLATEAU** – Stagnation of progression.

**POSITIVE ENERGY BALANCE** – When the amount of calories consumed exceeds the amount of calories expended. This is required for weight gain.

**POWER** – The product of force and velocity.

**PROGRESSIVE OVERLOAD** – A progressively increasing amount of stress placed on the body.

**PROTEIN BALANCE** – The ratio between protein synthesis and protein breakdown.

**PROTEIN BREAKDOWN** – The breakdown of proteins. This can contribute to a negative protein balance, thus causing muscle loss.

**PROTEIN SYNTHESIS** – The building of proteins. This contributes to a positive protein balance, which is necessary for muscle growth.

**REPETITION** – A repeated movement (i.e., lifting a weight in the same motion 10 times equates to 10 repetitions).

**REST INTERVAL** – The amount of time spent resting between sets.

**SET** – A grouping of repetitions performed without rest.

**STEADY-STATE CARDIO** – Aerobic training performed at a slow to moderate pace for long durations of time. Examples include jogging and moderate-intensity cycling.

**SUPERCOMPENSATION** – When the body rapidly adapts to an exercise program. This usually occurs following a period of rest, whereby the body adapts and becomes stronger from the training imposed on it prior to the rest period.

**TAPER PERIOD** – A systematic reduction in training volume designed to allow the athlete to "peak" in readiness for a competition.

**TESTOSTERONE** – An androgenic hormone primarily responsible for male characteristics. Can substantially increase muscle and strength when administered in high doses.

**TIME UNDER TENSION** – The amount of time a muscle is under strain during a set.

**TRAINING FREQUENCY** – Can refer to the amount of training sessions performed per week. In many cases, training frequency refers to the amount of times each muscle group is trained per week.

**TYPE I MUSCLE FIBER** – Known as a "slow twitch" muscle fiber, these are highly resistant to fatigue. However, they cannot produce as much force as type II muscle fibers.

**TYPE II MUSCLE FIBER** – Known as a "fast twitch" muscle fiber, these can generate high amounts of force, but they fatigue faster than type I muscle fibers.

**UNLOADING CYCLE** – Similar to a taper period, unloading cycles consist of planned reductions in training volume and/or intensity to promote recovery. While taper periods may last 1–4 weeks in duration, unloading cycles generally last 1 week.

**VOLUME** – The amount of sets multiplied by the amount of repetitions performed.

**VOLUME LOAD** – The amount of sets multiplied by the amount of repetitions multiplied by the load lifted.

Printed in Great Britain
by Amazon